HEART DISEASE IN MEN:

"Recognizing The Symptoms And Reducing Your Risk"

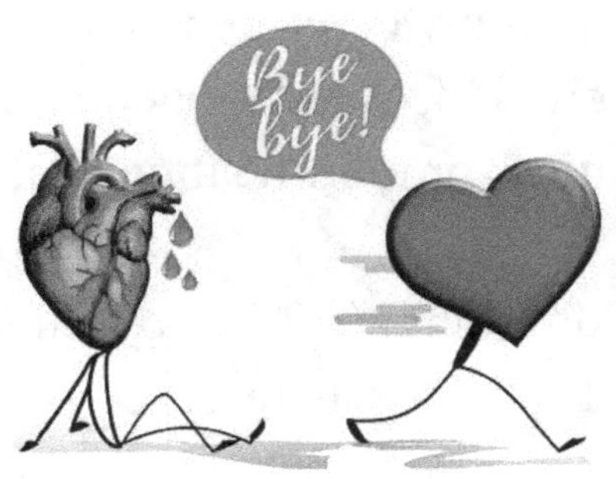

By Mercy Eunice

Copyright

Dedication

This book is dedicated to the many guys who have lost their lives prematurely due to heart disease and to their loved ones.

May this book serve as a guiding light for awareness, education, and action, enabling all of us to see the warning signals, lower our risk, and safeguard the health of our hearts.

Let's work together to stop this silent killer and work toward a day when heart disease is no longer the number one killer.

Heartfelt regards,

Mercy Eunice

Table of Contents

Introduction

The greatest cause of mortality for males globally is heart disease. Millions of men suffer from this silent killer, which often strikes without warning. Regardless of a man's lifestyle, family history, or general health, heart disease may attack at any age. Even yet, a lot of men wait until it's too late to detect the signs of heart disease.

In "Heart Disease in Men: Identifying the Signs and Lowering Your Risk," we delve into the heart disease realm and its effects on men's health. This book is a thorough handbook that arms readers with the information and resources they need to see the early warning symptoms of heart disease and take action to stop it from spreading.

Heart disease is a complicated disorder that may be brought on by a variety of lifestyle factors, including smoking, eating poorly, getting a little exercise, and stress. Environmental and genetic variables may also have an impact. Yet, men may take charge of their heart health and lower their risk of heart disease with the correct knowledge and techniques.

Also, it provides readers helpful guidance on how to lower their risk of heart disease via a balanced diet, consistent exercise, stress reduction, and other lifestyle adjustments. The book also goes over the need of getting medical help as soon as heart disease symptoms appear, since prompt treatment may significantly alter a man's prognosis.

The mission is to provide men with the information and tools they need to manage their heart health and lower their risk of developing heart disease. For men to live longer, healthier, and happier lives, we hope that this book will motivate them to take action and make life-changing changes.

Chapter 1: Understanding Heart Disease

What Is A Cardiac Condition?

The cardiovascular illness usually referred to as heart disease, is a broad term for several ailments that have an impact on the heart and blood arteries. It is a general phrase that covers some ailments, including heart failure, arrhythmias, and valve abnormalities.

The most prevalent kind of heart illness, coronary artery disease, happens when plaque, a fatty material, builds up in the blood channels supplying the heart with oxygen and nourishment, narrowing or blocking them. Angina, heart attacks, and other consequences may result from this.

Heart failure happens when the heart is unable to adequately pump blood, leading to fluid accumulation in the lungs and other bodily organs.

An abnormal cardiac rhythm is referred to as an arrhythmia, and it may make the heart beat too rapidly, too slowly, or irregularly.

When the heart valves do not close correctly or narrow excessively, they are said to have a valve problem, which may cause symptoms including exhaustion, chest discomfort, and shortness of breath.

Heart disease is a severe illness that poses a life-threatening risk, yet it is often preventable or manageable with the help of medicine, lifestyle modifications, and medical interventions.

How Do Guys With Heart Disease Fare?

Men's general health and quality of life may be significantly impacted by heart disease, which is a major health problem for males. Heart disease is the top cause of mortality for men in many nations throughout the globe and is more common in males than in women.

Men are more likely to get heart attacks as a result of having heart disease. A heart attack happens when the heart's blood supply is cut off, harming the heart muscle. Their health and welfare as well as their capacity to work and participate in other activities may be significantly impacted by this.

Men are also more likely to get heart failure as a result of having heart disease. Heart failure may cause symptoms including shortness of breath, exhaustion, and swelling in the legs and ankles when the heart can no longer adequately pump blood. Heart failure is more common in males than in women, and it may have a serious negative influence on a person's quality of life.

Heart disease may have long-term implications on men's health in addition to these acute ones. For instance, males who have heart illnesses are more likely to also experience diabetes, renal disease, and stroke. These ailments may need continuing treatment and care and have a negative influence on their health and well-being.

Lifestyle factors play a significant role in the increased risk of heart disease in males. In harmful activities including smoking, drinking alcohol, and eating a diet heavy in saturated fat and cholesterol, males are more prone than women to partake. Their risk of developing heart disease may rise as a result of these behaviors, which may also make it more challenging to manage the disease should it manifest.

High blood pressure, high cholesterol, diabetes, obesity, and a family history of heart disease are additional risk factors for heart disease in men. Men with these risk factors should take precautions to manage them, including altering their lifestyles, taking medications as directed, and closely observing their health.

Men's health is significantly affected by heart disease, which is a significant concern for their well-being. Men should be aware of their risk for heart disease and take action to lower it by changing their lifestyles, keeping an eye on their health, and, if necessary, seeing a doctor. Men can improve their general health and quality of life by taking proactive measures to prevent and manage heart disease.

The Many Forms Of Heart Illness

Heart disease is a general term for a number of ailments that have an impact on the heart and blood vessels. Heart disease comes in a variety of forms, each with its own causes, signs, and therapies.

The most prevalent kind of heart disease is called **Coronary Artery Disease (CAD),** and it happens when a buildup of plaque causes the arteries that carry blood to the heart to narrow or clog. This may result in heart attack, shortness of breath, and chest discomfort. High blood pressure, high cholesterol, smoking, and a family history of heart disease are risk factors for CAD.

Arrhythmia: An abnormal cardiac rhythm, which might be too slow, too rapid, or irregular, is referred to as an arrhythmia. This may result in symptoms including palpitations, lightheadedness, and fainting. Heart disease, adverse drug reactions, and electrolyte imbalances are just a few of the causes of arrhythmias.

Heart Failure: When the heart is unable to pump blood efficiently, fluid accumulates in the lungs and other bodily organs, leading to heart failure. This may result in symptoms including weariness, shortness of breath, and swelling in the ankles and legs. Heart failure may be brought on by a number of conditions, such as CAD, hypertension, and diabetes.

Cardiomyopathy: When the heart muscle is enlarged, thicker, or inflexible, it becomes more difficult for the heart to pump blood efficiently.

This may result in signs and symptoms include weariness, swelling in the ankles and legs, and breathing problems. Many variables, including heredity, viral infections, and alcohol misuse, might contribute to cardiomyopathy.

Heart Valve Disease: Heart valve disease is a condition in which the heart's valves do not close correctly or narrow excessively. Chest discomfort, exhaustion, and shortness of breath are a few symptoms that may result from this. Congenital flaws, infection, and age are only a few of the causes of heart valve dysfunction.

Heart problems that are apparent at birth are referred to as **Congenital Heart Disease**. They may include flaws in the heart's blood arteries, valves, or walls. Depending on the nature and degree of the problem, congenital heart disease may produce a variety of symptoms.

Peripheral Artery Disease (PAD): When plaque deposits constrict or block the arteries that provide blood to the legs, PAD develops.

Leg soreness and cramps may result from this, particularly while exercising. PAD raises the risk of heart attack and stroke and is a warning that a person may also have CAD.

A variety of illnesses that might harm the heart and blood arteries are included in the term "heart disease". Individuals may improve their overall heart health by taking actions to avoid and manage the many forms of heart disease and learning about its causes, symptoms, and treatments.

Heart Disease In Men: Causes And Risk Factors

Millions of individuals throughout the globe suffer from heart disease, and males are more likely than women to get the illness. Men's heart disease may be caused by a variety of factors, including lifestyle choices, underlying medical disorders, and genetic susceptibility.

Lifestyle Elements

Living a healthy lifestyle is one of the biggest risk factors for developing heart disease in males. Bad lifestyle decisions including smoking, binge drinking, being sedentary, and eating unhealthily may all raise the chance of getting heart disease. Smoking, in particular, destroys the lining of the arteries, raises blood pressure, and aids in the development of blood clots, making it a major contributor to heart disease in males. Similar to overdosing on alcohol, these conditions include heart failure, irregular pulse, and high blood pressure. Heart disease may also be brought on by a sedentary lifestyle and an unhealthily high-saturated-fat, trans-fat, salt, and sugar diet.

Health Conditions

The risk of heart disease in males might also be increased by certain medical disorders. Obesity, diabetes, high blood sugar, high cholesterol, and high blood pressure are all diseases that are directly related to the onset of heart disease.

Hypertension, another name for high blood pressure, raises the risk of heart attack and stroke and may damage the arteries. Similar to how narrowed arteries make it harder for blood to reach the heart, excessive cholesterol levels may lead to plaque development in the arteries. Diabetes may harm the blood vessels and nerves that regulate the heart, which increases the risk of heart disease. Obesity, or being significantly overweight, can raise the risk of heart disease because it places an additional burden on the heart and can result in the emergence of other health problems like high blood pressure and diabetes.

Genetic Propensity

Men's heart disease is largely caused by lifestyle choices and underlying medical conditions, but genetics also play a part. Men who have a history of heart disease in their families are more likely to get the disease themselves. Furthermore, some genetic conditions, like familial hypercholesterolemia, can raise cholesterol levels and raise the risk of heart disease.

Gender And Age

The last risk factors for heart disease in men are age and gender. As the risk of developing diseases like high blood pressure and high cholesterol rises with age, men over the age of 45 are more likely than younger men to develop heart disease. Men are also more likely than women to develop heart disease, particularly when they are younger. This is partially attributed to the fact that men are more likely to adopt unhealthy lifestyle habits like smoking and binge drinking.

Heart disease is a serious health issue that many men experience globally. Heart disease risk can be raised by lifestyle choices like smoking, binge drinking, being inactive all the time, and eating poorly. Additional risk factors include diseases like diabetes, high cholesterol, high blood pressure, and obesity. Men's heart disease can develop for a variety of reasons, including genetics, age, and gender. To prevent and manage heart disease in men, it is crucial to understand its causes and risk factors. You can also lower your risk of developing the disease by maintaining a healthy lifestyle and managing any underlying medical conditions.

Chapter 2: Recognizing the Symptoms

Common Signs Of Male Heart Disease

Millions of men throughout the globe suffer from the deadly medical illness known as heart disease. This disorder develops when the blood arteries supplying the heart constrict or get obstructed, which causes the heart's blood flow to diminish. As a consequence, men with heart disease might have a variety of symptoms, which can vary in severity depending on the depth of the blockage in the blood arteries. We will discuss the typical signs of heart disease in males in this long paragraph, such as weariness, shortness of breath, and chest discomfort.

Chest Ache

Chest discomfort, often known as angina, is one of the most prevalent signs of heart disease in males. When the heart does not get enough oxygenated blood, it might experience this kind of pain, which can feel tight or uncomfortable in the chest. In addition, the arms, neck, jaw, shoulder, or back may experience a radiating ache. Physical exertion or mental stress may cause chest discomfort, which is often eased by rest or medicine. Nevertheless, persistent chest discomfort and other symptoms like sweating, nausea, or shortness of breath might be signs of a heart attack and need immediate medical treatment.

Breath Control Issues

Another typical sign of heart disease in males is shortness of breath. Breathlessness or breathing difficulties resulting from the heart's inability to pump enough blood to fulfill the needs of the body. Men with heart disease may feel wheezing or coughing, as well as shortness of breath during exercise or rest. Chest discomfort, exhaustion, or swelling in the legs and ankles may also accompany shortness of breath.

Fatigue

Another typical sign of heart disease in men is fatigue or a sensation of weakness or exhaustion. This symptom may appear when the heart cannot pump enough blood to fulfill the body's energy requirements, resulting in a tired or worn-out sensation. Men with heart disease may get exhausted when engaging in physical activity or even at rest, and they may also have trouble sleeping or feel drained of energy. Other symptoms including shortness of breath, chest discomfort, or dizziness may also accompany the fatigue.

Extra Symptoms

Men with heart disease may have a variety of additional symptoms in addition to chest discomfort, breathlessness, and exhaustion. These symptoms may include dizziness or lightheadedness, nausea or vomiting, perspiration, palpitations, or a fast or irregular pulse. In addition to ankle and leg swelling, men with heart disease may also have fluid buildup in the tissues as a result of inadequate blood flow.

Males may have a variety of symptoms due to heart disease, a dangerous medical issue. Men who have heart disease often experience chest discomfort, shortness of breath, and exhaustion, but they might also have additional symptoms including nausea, dizziness, or swelling in their legs and ankles. It's important to seek medical care as soon as you notice any of these symptoms since fast diagnosis and treatment may lower the risk of problems and enhance results.

The Warning Indicators You Shouldn't Disregard

Knowing the symptoms of this lethal ailment is essential since heart disease is one of the major causes of mortality in men globally. Sadly, many men disregard these symptoms or misinterpret them, delaying diagnosis and treatment.

One of the most prevalent signs of heart disease in males is **Chest Pain Or Discomfort**. It often affects the middle of the chest and might feel pressing, squeezing, full, or burning. The arms, neck, jaw, or back may also experience a radiating ache. An indication of heart disease may be chest discomfort that worsens with rest but disappears after physical exertion or times of stress.

Breathlessness: Men with heart disease may feel short of breath, particularly while exercising or when lying down. There may be an accumulation of fluid in the lungs as a result of the heart's failure to pump enough blood to fulfill the body's requirements. Breathlessness that becomes worse over time might be an indication of heart failure.

Fatigue: Even after a full night's sleep or little effort, men with heart disease may experience particularly high levels of exhaustion. This results in a sense of weakness or lethargy because the heart is unable to pump enough blood to satisfy the body's requirements.

Dizziness or Fainting: Men with heart disease may feel dizziness or fainting, particularly after exercise or after standing up suddenly. Reduced blood flow to the brain or a dip in blood pressure might be to blame for this. A cardiac condition may potentially manifest as fainting or passing out.

Heart Palpitations or an Erratic Heartbeat are common in men with heart disease. This may have the effect of making your heart race, skip beats, or flutter. An arrhythmia, a disorder that affects the electrical system of the heart, may be the cause of an irregular heartbeat.

Swelling: The legs, ankles, or feet of men with heart disease may enlarge. This results from an accumulation of fluid in the body, which happens when the heart cannot efficiently pump blood.

Men with heart disease may have **Nausea, Vomiting,** or **Indigestion**, particularly if they also have other risk factors including diabetes, high blood pressure, or high cholesterol. Reduced blood supply to the digestive tract may be the cause of these symptoms.

Men with heart disease could have **Cold Sweats**, particularly while they're exercising or under stress. This could be a result of the body's reaction to less blood flowing to the skin.

Heart disease is a primary cause of mortality in males throughout the globe, making it crucial to be aware of its warning symptoms. Men should not disregard the warning indications of heart disease such as chest pain or discomfort, shortness of breath, exhaustion, dizziness or fainting, irregular heartbeat, swelling, nausea or indigestion, and cold sweats.

How To Recognize The Signs Of Heart Disease From Those Of Other Illnesses

If not identified and treated early, heart disease is a severe ailment that may result in life-threatening consequences. Yet, since some of its symptoms often overlap with those of other medical disorders, it can be difficult to discern between heart disease and other medical issues.

Chest Pain or Discomfort: While chest discomfort is often a sign of heart disease, it may also be brought on by other medical diseases including acid reflux, pneumonia, or torn muscles. Heart-related chest pain often occurs in the middle of the chest and may feel like pressure, squeezing fullness, or a burning feeling. This is the main distinction between chest pain from heart disease and chest pain from other causes. The arms, neck, jaw, or back may also experience a radiating ache. An indication of heart disease may be chest discomfort that worsens with rest but disappears after physical exertion or times of stress.

Breathlessness: Breathlessness is another typical heart disease symptom, although it may also be brought on by other illnesses including asthma, pneumonia, or Chronic Obstructive Pulmonary Disease (COPD). The main distinction between shortness of breath brought on by heart disease and other reasons is that the former often occurs when laying down or engaging in physical activity. There can be a cough or wheezing as well. Breathlessness that becomes worse over time might be an indication of heart failure.

Fatigue: While it might be a sign of heart disease, fatigue can also be brought on by other medical illnesses including anemia, depression, or thyroid issues. The main distinction between weariness from heart disease and other causes is that the latter is often accompanied by additional symptoms like shortness of breath or chest discomfort. It could also become more noticeable when you strain yourself physically.

Dizziness or Lightheadedness: While dizziness or fainting may be a sign of heart disease, it can also be brought on by other medical disorders such as dehydration, low blood sugar, or anemia. The main distinction between dizziness or fainting brought on by heart disease and other reasons is that the former often happens during or after exercise. Other symptoms, such as shortness of breath or chest discomfort, may also be present.

An **Irregular Heartbeat** or **Palpitations** may be a sign of heart disease, but they can also be brought on by other health issues including worry, coffee usage, or thyroid issues. The main distinction between an irregular heartbeat caused by heart disease and those caused by other conditions is that heart palpitations frequently come with additional symptoms like chest pain or shortness of breath. These could also happen while you're exercising or under stress.

Swelling: Although swelling in the legs, ankles, or feet might be a sign of heart disease, it can also be brought on by other illnesses such as renal, liver, or blood clot disease. The main distinction between swelling brought on by heart illness and edema brought on by other conditions is that heart-related swelling often affects both legs and is more apparent at night. Other symptoms, such as weariness or shortness of breath, may also be present.

In addition to being a sign of heart disease, **Nausea** and **Indigestion** may also be brought on by other illnesses such as food poisoning, gastroesophageal reflux disease (GERD), and stomach viruses. The main distinction between indigestion or nausea brought on by heart disease and other reasons is that heart-related symptoms often coexist with other symptoms like shortness of breath or chest discomfort. These could also happen while you're exercising or under stress.

When Should You Get Medical Help?

Heart disease is a critical disorder that, if neglected, may have fatal effects. Heart failure, arrhythmias, coronary artery disease, and issues with the heart valves are just a few of the disorders that go under the umbrella term "heart disease," which affects both the heart and blood arteries.

To get a thorough diagnosis and course of therapy for heart disease, it's crucial to seek medical help as soon as possible. When symptoms appear, which might vary depending on the exact problem, many people may not know they have heart disease. Chest pain or discomfort, shortness of breath, exhaustion, dizziness, and fainting are some typical signs of heart disease.

It's crucial to get medical help immediately away if you develop any of these symptoms. When it comes to heart disease, it is always better to be safe than sorry, even if the symptoms are minor. Heart disease may sometimes advance quickly, resulting in a heart attack or stroke.

High blood pressure, high cholesterol, smoking, diabetes, obesity, and a family history of the illness are some of the variables that raise the risk of heart disease. It is crucial to take charge of your heart health if you have any of these risk factors, so talk to your doctor about them. Your doctor can assist you in creating a strategy that includes both lifestyle modifications and medicines to lower your risk of developing heart disease.

It's important to schedule regular check-ups with your doctor to monitor your heart health in addition to obtaining medical assistance for heart disease symptoms. To evaluate how well your heart is working, your doctor could advise tests like an electrocardiogram (ECG), echocardiography, or stress test.

If you have heart disease, it's crucial to adhere to your doctor's advice on medication and lifestyle modifications. In addition to dietary and activity modifications, this may also include the use of drugs to treat symptoms and lower the likelihood of problems.

In certain circumstances, more intrusive treatments for heart disease, such as angioplasty or bypass surgery, may be required. It is crucial to explore the advantages and disadvantages of these treatments with your doctor since they may be quite successful but also carry hazards.

To sum up, heart disease is a dangerous issue that has to be treated right away. If you see any heart disease symptoms, you should consult a doctor straight once. Talk to your doctor about strategies to lower your risk and keep an eye on your heart health if you have other risk factors for heart disease. You may lower your chance of issues and live a healthier, happier life by taking good care of your heart.

Chapter 3: Diagnostic Tests

The Many Heart Disease Diagnostic Procedures

Depending on the precise condition and symptoms a patient is exhibiting, the diagnosis of heart disease may need several different tests. Electrocardiograms (ECGs), echocardiograms, stress tests, cardiac catheterization, and coronary angiography are some of the main tests used to identify heart illness.

A quick test to gauge the electrical activity of the heart is an **Electrocardiogram (ECG).** Electrodes are positioned on the skin of the chest, arms, and legs during a painless operation. The test normally just takes a few minutes and may assist in identifying cardiac rhythm irregularities, coronary artery blockages, and other conditions that can result in heart disease.

Another non-invasive diagnostic that produces pictures of the heart using sound waves is **Echocardiography**. It may provide details about the heart's dimensions and physical characteristics, as well as how efficiently it pumps blood. This test may also be used to find blood clots, heart valve abnormalities, and other conditions that might aggravate heart disease.

A Stress Test is a procedure that assesses how well the heart works under stress. A patient will be asked to walk on a treadmill or ride a stationary bike during a stress test while their blood pressure and heart rate are being watched. This test may be able to find coronary artery blockages that would not be noticeable otherwise.

Cardiac Catheterization is a more intrusive examination that entails threading a tiny tube (a catheter) up to the heart via a blood artery in the groin or arm. The location and degree of any blockages in the coronary arteries, as well as other pertinent information, may be determined by this examination. Moreover, it may be used to collect blood and cardiac tissue, as well as to gauge the pressure within the heart.

A particular dye is injected into the coronary arteries during a heart catheterization procedure known as **Coronary Angiography**. Afterward, X-ray pictures are obtained to show how the arteries and heart pump blood. This test may aid in pinpointing the location and degree of coronary artery blockages, which is helpful for therapy planning.

Nuclear Imaging Studies, such as a PET scan or a Single-Photon Emission Computed Tomography (SPECT) scan, and magnetic resonance imaging (MRI) are further procedures that may be used to identify cardiac problems. These exams may provide precise pictures of the heart and blood arteries and can show where there is inadequate blood flow or cardiac muscle injury.

In addition to these tests, a patient's medical history, physical exam, and other criteria, such as age and risk factors for heart disease, may also be examined when reaching a diagnosis. After a heart disease diagnosis, a patient may explore their treatment choices with a healthcare professional. These options may include making lifestyle adjustments, taking medicines, or having treatments like angioplasty or bypass surgery.

A variety of tests may be done to identify cardiac disease, based on the patient's particular state and present symptoms. These tests may aid in the identification of coronary artery blockages, abnormal cardiac rhythms, and other conditions that may be associated with heart disease. Patients may lower their risk of problems and live healthier, longer lives by recognizing and treating heart disease early.

What To Anticipate During Diagnostic Exams

While having diagnostic testing for heart disease, it is common to feel apprehensive or unclear about what to anticipate. Nevertheless, addressing some of these worries and ensuring a more pleasant experience may be accomplished by being aware of what the exams include and how to prepare. This is a full overview of what to anticipate during some of the most popular diagnostic tests for heart disease.

An **Electrocardiogram (ECG)** examines the electrical activity of the heart and is a non-invasive diagnostic. Little electrodes are affixed to the skin of the arms, legs, and chest during an ECG. The electrodes are attached to a machine that records the heart's electrical impulses. There is no need to fast or alter your normal routine before the test, which typically lasts 10 minutes.

Echocardiogram: An echocardiogram is a non-invasive test that utilizes sound waves to produce pictures of the heart. A technician will apply a gel to the patient's chest before gliding a tiny wand-like instrument (the transducer) over the skin to do an echocardiogram. Images that may be seen on a screen are produced when sound waves from the transducer are reflected off the heart and travel through the body. The test normally takes around 30-60 minutes, and there is no need to fast or adjust your routine before the test.

Stress Test: A stress test is a procedure that assesses how well the heart functions under stress. A patient will be asked to walk on a treadmill or ride a stationary bike during a stress test while their blood pressure and heart rate are being watched. The exam normally takes around 30-60 minutes, and patients should wear comfortable clothes and shoes suited for the activity. Also, it is advised to wait at least 4 hours before the test to eat or drink anything other than water.

Heart Catheterization: Cardiac catheterization is a more intrusive procedure that entails threading a tiny tube (a catheter) up to the heart via a blood artery in the arm or groin. Patients often get a sedative before the surgery and local anesthesia to numb the region where the catheter is implanted. The heart and blood arteries are seen using X-rays and a specific dye. To prevent bleeding at the catheter site, patients must remain motionless for many hours after the treatment. The test typically lasts between 30 and 60 minutes.

Coronary Angiography: A kind of cardiac catheterization known as coronary angiography involves injecting a particular dye into the coronary arteries. Afterward, X-ray pictures are obtained to show how the arteries and heart pump blood. To prevent bleeding at the catheter site, patients must remain motionless for many hours after the treatment. The test typically lasts between 30 and 60 minutes.

Nuclear Imaging Tests: Using a tiny quantity of radioactive material, nuclear imaging tests, such as a **Positron Emission Tomography (PET)** scan or a **Single-Photon Emission Computed**

Tomography (SPECT) scan, provide pictures of the heart and blood arteries. The radioactive substance is administered to patients either intravenously or by gas inhalation. Patients may be requested to refrain from eating or drinking anything other than water for several hours before the test, which typically lasts 30 to 60 minutes.

Magnetic Resonance Imaging (MRI): Magnetic resonance imaging (MRI) is a non-invasive procedure that produces precise pictures of the heart and blood arteries using a strong magnetic field and radio waves. Patients recline on a table that slides into a big tube-shaped machine during an MRI. Patients must remain motionless and lay flat for the duration of the test, which typically lasts 30 to 60 minutes.

The complexity and invasiveness of heart disease diagnostic tests might vary. It's critical to comprehend the rationale behind each exam as well as what to anticipate from the process. It's also crucial to adhere to any preparation guidelines provided by your doctor, such as fasting or avoiding certain drugs. Some tests, like ECGs and echocardiograms, are non-invasive and very straightforward, but others, like cardiac catheterization and nuclear imaging tests, may be more intrusive and need more preparation.

Tips For Getting Ready For Diagnostic Exams

It is possible to assure accurate findings and a more pleasant experience by preparing for diagnostic testing. It is crucial to adhere to any instructions provided by your healthcare practitioner since various tests may have different preparation needs. *Here are some general pointers for being ready for diagnostic exams:*

Following the test, you may be required to fast for a certain period before the process. This suggests that you should just consume water. To get accurate results, be sure to carefully follow these directions.

A list of your current medications, including over-the-counter medicines and dietary supplements, should be brought to the test. This might assist your doctor in determining if any drugs need to be discontinued or altered before the test.

Put on comfortable attire and exercise-appropriate shoes while doing exams like the stress test. Since they might affect the test, avoid wearing jewelry or clothes with metal buttons or zippers.

Come early to enable time for check-in and any required documentation at the testing location. Also, this may lessen tension and stress.

Talk to your healthcare practitioner if you have any questions or concerns regarding the test. Do not be afraid to ask your healthcare provider any questions. They may provide you with further details about the test's objectives, what to anticipate throughout the process, and any risks or side effects that could occur.

Observe any further detailed instructions: There may be additional particular directions to follow, such as halting the use of certain drugs or abstaining from caffeine, depending on the test. To get accurate results, be sure to carefully follow these directions.

Bring a support person: You may wish to bring a support person with you to the process, depending on the test and your particular requirements. This may provide solace and certainty during the procedure.

Preparing for diagnostic testing includes adhering to any particular directions provided by your healthcare professional, being upfront about any worries or inquiries, and taking precautions to make the procedure as pleasant as possible. By adhering to these recommendations, you may aid in ensuring accurate outcomes and efficient heart disease and other cardiac disorders diagnosis and treatment.

Understanding Test Results

Understanding the precise test being utilized as well as what normal and abnormal findings may signify is necessary for interpreting test results for cardiac disease. *In general, consider the following when evaluating test results*:

Understand The Test's Objective: Various tests are used to identify various forms of heart disease, therefore it's crucial to be aware of this. An echocardiogram, for instance, may be used to assess the anatomy and function of the heart, while an ECG can be used to identify arrhythmias.

Recognize Usual Findings: Before interpreting test results, it's critical to recognize typical outcomes for the particular test being conducted. This may change based on elements including age, gender, and general health.

Look For Trends: Rather than concentrating exclusively on individual numbers when interpreting test results, it is vital to search for trends and patterns. An ECG, for instance, may sometimes reveal irregular cardiac rhythms that, if they persist over time, may be serious.

Examine The Patient's General State Of Health: Test findings should always be evaluated in light of the patient's general state of health. For instance, compared to a patient without a history of cardiac issues, a patient with established heart disease may have more serious implications for negative exercise stress test findings.

Speak With A Medical Professional: Deciphering test findings may be challenging and takes extensive expertise. It is crucial to speak with a medical professional who can interpret the test findings and explain their importance in light of the patient's overall health.

Based on the results, they may also suggest any required further tests or treatments.

Ask Questions: Don't be afraid to ask your healthcare practitioner for further details if you have any queries or worries regarding the test findings. They may give extra information and assist you to understand what the findings signify for your health.

Knowing the particular test being performed, being aware of what normal and abnormal findings can mean, and taking into account the patient's general health are all necessary when interpreting test results for cardiac disease. Asking questions and seeking advice from a healthcare professional may assist ensure that test findings are correctly interpreted and that the right follow-up treatment is provided.

Chapter 4: Reducing Your Risk

Adapt Your Lifestyle To Lower Your Risk Of Heart Disease

While heart disease is one of the top causes of mortality in the world, many instances may be avoided by changing one's lifestyle. Healthy lifestyle choices like regular exercise, a balanced diet, and stress management may lower your risk of heart disease and enhance your cardiovascular health in general. *The following lifestyle modifications may be performed to lower the chance of developing heart disease*:

Work Out Frequently: Maintaining heart health requires regular physical exercise. Strive for at least 150 minutes of moderate-intensity activity each week, such as brisk walking or cycling. Strength training activities should be used at least twice a week to assist enhance cardiovascular health.

Keep A Healthy Diet: Cholesterol, blood pressure and weight are all risk factors for heart disease. A nutritious diet may help decrease these numbers. Be sure to emphasize eating a variety of fruits, vegetables, whole grains, lean protein sources, and healthy fats like nuts and seeds. Reduce your intake of added sugars, saturated fats, and trans fats.

Control Your Stress: Heart disease may be exacerbated by ongoing stress. Use stress-relieving methods like yoga, deep breathing, or meditation. Take part in leisure pursuits and activities that make you happy and relaxed.

Stop Smoking: Smoking is a significant risk factor for heart disease, and giving up is one of the most effective ways to lower your risk. To help you stop smoking, ask your friends, family, or medical experts for assistance.

Reduce Your Alcohol Intake since excessive drinking raises your risk of heart disease and other illnesses. If you prefer to consume alcohol, keep your consumption to moderate levels, which for women is one drink per day and for males is two drinks per day.

Maintain Healthy Blood Pressure And Cholesterol Levels: Two significant risk factors for heart disease are high blood pressure and high cholesterol. The risk of heart disease may be decreased with routine blood pressure and cholesterol treatment. A good diet and regular exercise may help regulate these risks, as can prescribed medications.

Obesity is a risk factor for heart disease, so **keep your weight in check**. Heart disease risk may be lowered by maintaining a healthy weight via a wholesome diet and frequent exercise.

Establishing healthy lifestyle practices including consistent exercise, a balanced diet, stress management, giving up smoking, consuming little to no alcohol, managing blood pressure and cholesterol levels, and keeping a healthy weight will help lower the risk of heart disease. Consistently making little adjustments may have a big impact on your cardiovascular health and general well-being.

Advice On Nutrition And Diet

A heart-healthy diet may be very helpful for men with heart disease in treating their illness and lowering their chance of developing new cardiovascular problems. *For males with heart disease, the following food and nutrition advice is provided:*

A heart-healthy diet should include complete, nutrient-dense foods, such as fruits, vegetables, whole grains, lean meats, and healthy fats. These foods are bursting with antioxidants, vitamins, and minerals that may protect the heart and enhance cardiovascular health in general.

Reduce your intake of processed and high-fat meals: These items, such as fast food, fried foods, and sweets, may raise your blood pressure, raise your cholesterol, and make you gain weight, all of which are risk factors for heart disease. The heart's health may be improved by limiting certain foods.

Including omega-3 fatty acids in your diet: Studies have shown that these fats may protect the heart. Fatty seafood like salmon and tuna as well as flaxseed, chia seeds, and walnuts are sources of omega-3s.

Choose lean proteins: Protein helps you feel full and helps you retain muscle mass. Unfortunately, certain protein sources may include a lot of saturated fat, which raises the risk of heart disease. Choose lean proteins like those found in fish, poultry, and plant-based sources like beans and lentils.

Reduce your salt intake: High blood pressure, a key risk factor for heart disease, may be a result of a high sodium diet. Improve heart health by reducing sodium consumption by avoiding processed meals, using less salt while cooking, and selecting low-sodium substitutes.

Be hydrated: Dehydration may increase the risk of high blood pressure and strain the heart. To keep hydrated and maintain general cardiovascular health, make an effort to drink enough water throughout the day.

Exercise portion control since eating too much may lead to weight gain, which increases your chance of developing heart disease. Using smaller plates, calculating meal portions, and being aware of your hunger and fullness signals are all ways to practice portion management and support a healthy weight.

Partnering with a licensed dietitian may help men with heart disease create a personalized dietary plan that suits their particular requirements and interests. Men who want to make long-lasting dietary and lifestyle changes might benefit from the instruction and assistance that a nutritionist can provide.

A heart-healthy diet for men with heart disease should prioritize whole, nutrient-dense foods, minimize processed and high-fat foods, including omega-3 fatty acids, select lean proteins, limit sodium intake, maintain hydration, practice portion control, and collaborate with a registered dietitian for individualized advice and support. Men with heart disease may improve their overall cardiovascular health and lower their risk of further cardiovascular events by adopting minor, consistent adjustments to their diet and lifestyle.

Workout Guidelines For Heart Disease In Males

For men, exercise is a crucial part of managing the cardiac disease. Frequent exercise may lower the risk of future cardiovascular events, enhance the overall quality of life, and improve cardiovascular health. To ensure that they exercise safely and efficiently, men with heart disease must adhere to particular exercise instructions.

Contact your doctor: Men with heart problems should speak with their doctor before beginning an exercise program to be sure it is safe for them to do so. They may need a stress test or other diagnostic procedures, depending on the severity of their cardiac condition, to establish the right amount of activity.

Men with heart disease should begin their exercise routine gradually and build up to a higher level of intensity over time. By doing so, you can protect yourself from harm and make sure your heart can withstand the added strain. Starting with low-impact workouts like walking or cycling is a smart idea.

Strive for moderate-intensity exercise: Men with heart disease should pursue moderate-intensity exercise, which is characterized as a conversation-friendly activity that elevates the heart rate and breathing rate.

Exercises that fall under the category of moderate intensity include swimming, dancing, cycling, and brisk walking.

Including resistance exercise: Strength training, also known as resistance training, may assist to increase muscular strength and endurance, which can enhance cardiovascular health. Men with heart disease should start with modest weights and high repetitions when incorporating resistance training into their fitness regimen.

Men with heart disease should keep an eye on their symptoms while they are exercising. They should stop exercising and see their doctor if they feel chest discomfort, shortness of breath, lightheadedness, or dizziness.

Men with heart disease should strive to exercise often to gain the advantages of exercise. A minimum of 150 minutes of moderate-intensity exercise each week, distributed over at least three days, is advised by the American Heart Association.

Exercise in a safe setting: Men with heart disease should exercise in a safe environment. They should exercise inside or in more temperate temperatures since extreme heat or cold might strain the heart even more.

Consider working with a qualified personal trainer: It may be advantageous to work with a qualified personal trainer who has expertise in training people with heart disease. Men with heart disease may exercise safely and efficiently with the aid of a personal trainer who can provide direction and encouragement.

Men with heart disease should seek medical advice before beginning an exercise regimen, begin gradually, aim for moderate-intensity exercise, incorporate resistance training, monitor symptoms, exercise frequently, be aware of the environment, and think about hiring a certified personal trainer. Men with heart disease may improve their cardiovascular health and lower their risk of further cardiovascular events by adhering to these exercise suggestions.

How To Control Anxiety And Stress

Although stress and worry are normal parts of daily life, they may harm our health, especially the cardiovascular system. It is generally known that there is a link between chronic stress and heart disease, with chronic stress raising the chance of developing heart disease and worsening pre-existing heart diseases. A healthy heart may be maintained by controlling stress and lowering anxiety. *The following are some techniques for controlling stress and lowering anxiety:*

Locate the causes of stress in your life and make an effort to avoid or reduce them, if at all feasible. Try to alter how you react to them if you can't avoid them. This may include discovering new coping mechanisms or asking for assistance from close relatives, close friends, or a mental health professional.

Use relaxation methods: These methods may help you feel calmer and more at ease by reducing tension and anxiety. Deep breathing, gradual muscular relaxation, guided visualization, and meditation are a few examples of relaxation methods.

Exercise regularly: An exercise is a terrific approach to reducing stress and enhancing cardiovascular health in general. Endorphins are naturally occurring mood enhancers that are released during physical exercise and may help lower anxiety and despair.

Sleep is crucial for both physical and mental health, so get plenty of it. Lack of sleep may worsen cardiovascular health and raise levels of stress and anxiety. Strive for 7-8 hours of sleep every night, minimum.

Consume a nutritious diet: A nutritious diet may help lower stress and anxiety as well as enhance cardiovascular health. Limit processed and high-fat foods and strive for a diet heavy in fruits, vegetables, whole grains, lean protein, and healthy fats.

Cultivate mindfulness: Mindfulness entails being present at the moment without passing judgment on it. Yoga, tai chi, and other mindfulness exercises may help lessen stress and anxiety while fostering emotions of tranquility and well-being.

Get assistance: If you often feel stressed or anxious, you may want to think about getting help from a mental health expert. You may acquire new coping mechanisms and lessen the harmful effects of stress on your health via therapy.

Controlling stress and lowering anxiety are crucial stages in preserving a healthy heart. Identifying causes of stress, using relaxation techniques, exercising often, getting enough sleep, eating a nutritious diet, practicing mindfulness, and having support are all methods for managing stress and anxiety. You may increase your general well-being and lower your chance of getting heart disease by implementing these techniques into your everyday life.

Chapter 5: Treatment Options

Drugs For The Treatment Of Heart Problems

The prevention, diagnosis, and treatment of heart disease all include the use of medications. Several drugs may be used to treat symptoms, reduce risk factors, and avoid heart disease consequences. *Following are some typical drugs for treating cardiac disease*:

Statins: A class of drugs called statins is used to reduce blood cholesterol levels. Statins may aid in lowering the risk of heart attack and stroke. Elevated cholesterol is a significant risk factor for heart disease.

Beta-blockers: A family of drugs known as beta blockers are used to treat conditions such as high blood pressure, heart failure, and certain types of irregular heartbeat. They function by lowering the heart's workload and heart rate.

ACE Inhibitors: ACE inhibitors are a class of drugs used to treat heart failure and excessive blood pressure. They function by allowing the blood arteries to relax and lighten the burden on the heart.

Calcium Channel Blockers: A family of drugs known as calcium channel blockers is used to treat excessive blood pressure and certain cardiac rhythm problems. They relieve the pressure on the heart by relaxing the blood arteries.

Antiplatelet Agents: Drugs used to stop blood clots from developing include antiplatelet agents. Those who have experienced a heart attack, stroke or another kind of cardiovascular event are often given them.

Anticoagulants: Drugs that stop the formation of blood clots are known as anticoagulants. Those with atrial fibrillation or other cardiac diseases that raise the risk of blood clots are often administered them.

Diuretics: A class of drugs called diuretics is used to treat heart failure and excessive blood pressure. They function by eliminating extra fluid from the body, which may lessen the strain on the heart.

As a medicine, **nitroglycerin** is used to relieve chest discomfort (angina). It works by widening the blood arteries and boosting heart-related blood flow.

Digoxin is a drug that is used to treat some cardiac rhythm problems as well as heart failure. It works by reducing heart rate and boosting the force of each heartbeat.

Vasodilators: Drugs that relax blood vessels and improve blood flow are known as vasodilators. For those who have heart failure or excessive blood pressure, they are often recommended.

Surgery To Treat Heart Disease

Surgery may be advised when lifestyle modifications and prescription drugs are insufficient to control or treat heart disease. Depending on the nature and severity of the ailment, a variety of surgical treatments may be employed to treat heart disease. *These are a few typical surgeries for treating heart disease:*

The surgical treatment known as **Coronary Artery Bypass Grafting (CABG)** is performed to relieve blockages in the coronary arteries, which carry blood to the heart muscle. With the surgery, a blood vessel from another region of the body is taken and used to bypass the coronary artery blockage, letting blood flow to the heart more easily.

Treatment for blockages in the coronary arteries using **Angioplasties And Stenting** are two minimally invasive procedures. A little balloon is inflated during the surgery to open up the blocked artery and increase blood flow. To assist keep the artery open, a stent (a little mesh tube) is often inserted inside it.

Heart Valve Replacement Or Repair: The surgical operation of heart valve replacement or repair is performed to correct issues with the heart's valves. A broken valve may be repaired or replaced with an artificial valve during the process.

Aneurysm Repair is a surgical treatment used to address aneurysms (weak areas) in the blood artery walls of the heart. To strengthen the vessel and stop it from rupturing, a surgeon may insert a graft (a tube formed of synthetic material) during the surgery.

Heart Transplant: A surgical procedure called a heart transplant is done to treat advanced heart failure. A damaged heart is taken out during the process and replaced with a healthy heart from a donor.

Maze Procedure: A surgical treatment for the management of atrial fibrillation (an irregular heart rhythm). To reroute the electrical impulses that produce the erratic beat, a surgeon fashions a pattern of scar tissue in the upper chambers of the heart during the surgery.

Surgery has dangers, therefore it's crucial to keep in mind that it should only be considered when the advantages may exceed the risks. The kind of treatment, as well as individual characteristics like age and general health, might affect recovery durations and results.

Adapting Your Lifestyle To Support Your Therapy

Making changes to one's lifestyle is crucial for treating and controlling heart disease. Making certain adjustments to your everyday routine may assist your treatment plan and enhance your overall heart health, even while drugs and surgical treatments can be beneficial in addressing the issue. *The following lifestyle changes may assist in the management of heart disease:*

Stop Smoking: Smoking increases your chances of developing heart disease and may make any heart issues you already have worse. The risk of heart disease may be decreased, and general heart health can be improved, by quitting smoking. Consult your healthcare physician to learn about smoking cessation techniques.

Keep A Healthy Weight since it lowers your chance of developing heart disease. This risk may be decreased by maintaining a healthy weight with a balanced diet and frequent exercise. See a qualified dietician or member of the medical profession for advice on healthy weight control.

Consume A Heart-healthy Diet: A diet reduced in cholesterol, salt, and saturated and trans fats may assist to enhance heart health. Eat a mix of fruits, vegetables, whole grains, lean meats, and healthy fats like those in nuts and fish as your main focus.

Frequent Physical Exercise may help lower the risk of heart disease and enhance heart health. At least 150 minutes per week of moderate-intensity exercises, such as brisk walking, cycling, or swimming, should be your goal.

Control Your Stress: Heart disease may worsen and develop as a result of stress. Deep breathing, yoga, and other stress-reduction techniques may help lower stress levels and enhance overall heart health.

Reduce Your Alcohol Intake since excessive alcohol use raises your chance of developing heart disease. If you decide to consume alcohol, do so sparingly. One drink per day for women and two for men is the maximum amount that the American Heart Association advises.

Get Enough Sleep: Heart disease may develop and worsen as a result of insufficient sleep. To maintain heart health, aim for 7-8 hours of sleep each night.

It is vital to consult with a healthcare physician before making any big changes to your lifestyle, particularly if you have a pre-existing cardiac issue. A healthcare professional may advise you on safe and practical lifestyle changes that will complement your treatment plan and enhance your general heart health. You may actively participate in the prevention, treatment, and management of heart disease by making certain adjustments to your daily schedule and way of life.

How To Handle Heart Disease Complications

Several complications can arise from heart disease, which is a serious condition. It is crucial to be aware of these complications so that you can take action to manage them. They can range in severity from minor to life-threatening. Here are some strategies for controlling heart disease complications:

Arrhythmia: An irregular heartbeat is a condition known as arrhythmia. Shortness of breath, dizziness, and palpitations are possible side effects. Arrhythmia may be treated with drugs or actions that control the beating of the heart. It's crucial to get medical help if you experience arrhythmia symptoms.

Heart Attack: When the blood supply to the heart is cut off, the heart muscle suffers damage and a heart attack takes place. Medication or surgery to reestablish blood flow to the heart may be used as a treatment for a heart attack. If you experience heart attack symptoms like chest pain or discomfort, shortness of breath, or lightheadedness, it's critical to get emergency medical help.

When the heart cannot pump enough blood to meet the demands of the body, **Heart Failure** occurs. Medication, lifestyle changes, and surgery may all be used as heart failure treatments. Working closely with a healthcare professional is crucial for managing heart failure and avoiding problems.

Stroke: When the blood supply to the brain is cut off, brain cells are damaged, and a stroke results. Medications or surgical methods to reestablish blood flow to the brain may be used in stroke treatment. If you suffer stroke symptoms like abrupt weakness, numbness, or tingling on one side of your body, difficulty speaking or comprehending speech, or sudden vision changes, it's critical to get immediate medical help.

Peripheral Artery Disease: Peripheral artery disease is a narrowing or blocking of the arteries that provide blood to the legs and feet. Medication, dietary changes, or surgical techniques to reestablish blood flow to the damaged region may all be used as forms of treatment.

Pulmonary Embolism: A blood clot that enters the lungs and obstructs blood flow is known as a pulmonary embolism. The use of drugs or other treatments to dissolve the clot and stop new clots from forming may be part of the treatment.

Heart disease may cause other problems including high blood pressure, high cholesterol, and diabetes in addition to these side effects. It is possible to reduce the risk of problems and boost overall heart health by managing these disorders with medication, lifestyle changes, and routine doctor visits.

Working closely with a healthcare professional is crucial while managing heart disease problems. You may help avoid problems and enhance general heart health by adhering to a treatment plan and changing your lifestyle.

Chapter 6: Living with Heart Disease

Managing The Psychological And Emotional Repercussions Of Heart Disease

Being told you have heart disease may change your life and have a variety of emotional and psychological impacts. Heart disease patients often struggle with emotions of worry, despair, dread, and uncertainty. It may be difficult to deal with the emotional and psychological impacts of heart disease, but some methods might be useful.

Get support: You can manage the emotional and psychological repercussions of heart disease by speaking with family members, friends, and medical professionals. You could also think about joining a support group or getting professional assistance for your mental health.

Remain Informed: You might feel more in control and less concerned by being more knowledgeable about your situation. To learn more about your disease and your treatment choices, ask your healthcare physician for information and resources.

Use relaxation methods: Deep breathing, meditation, and yoga are all relaxation methods that may help you feel less stressed and anxious. Both at home and in a group situation, these strategies are effective.

Exercise: Physical exercise has been shown to help decrease stress and enhance mood. Speak with your healthcare practitioner about safe exercise alternatives that are suitable for your situation.

Keep a healthy diet: Eating healthfully may assist to promote overall well-being and heart health. Creating a meal plan that is suitable for your condition would need working with a licensed dietitian or other healthcare professionals.

Reduce your use of alcohol and cigarettes since both may increase the emotional and psychological consequences of heart disease and have a detrimental impact on your heart's health.

Maintaining medication compliance is important because certain drugs used to treat heart disease may have negative effects on behavior and mental well-being. Manage your prescriptions and keep an eye out for any adverse effects in collaboration with your healthcare practitioner.

It's important to keep in mind that overcoming the emotional and psychological impacts of heart disease is a lengthy journey. Seeking the assistance of a mental health expert is crucial if you are displaying signs of anxiety or despair. It is feasible to manage the emotional and psychological impacts of heart disease and enhance general well-being with the correct assistance and tools.

How To Maintain Motivation To Alter Your Way Of Life

It may be difficult to adjust one's lifestyle to promote heart health, and it's typical to struggle with motivation and sticking with new routines. But, some tactics might support your commitment to making long-term improvements and help you remain motivated.

Establish precise, attainable objectives: Achieving precise, attainable goals may keep you motivated and focused. Divide more difficult objectives into smaller, more achievable stages and acknowledge each accomplishment along the way.

Find a system of support: Be in the company of individuals who will support and motivate your attempts to improve your way of life. These might include close relatives, close friends, medical professionals, or a support group.

Maintain a progress log: Keeping a progress log helps keep you inspired and provides you with a visual depiction of your accomplishments. Tracking physical activity, food, and nutrition, as well as medication compliance, are some examples of this.

Employ encouraging language to yourself: Good self-talk may make you feel more motivated and confident. Employ affirmations like "I can accomplish this" or "I am capable of making good changes" to help you stay optimistic.

Reward yourself: Rewarding yourself for reaching milestones may inspire and support good behavior. This can include treating yourself to a special activity, item, or experience.

Making lifestyle changes fun may help them seem less like a chore and more like a rewarding experience. This can be done by finding entertaining hobbies and nutritious meals. Try out new recipes, engage in various types of exercise, and discover exciting methods to make healthy choices.

Envision success: You may visualize success and increase motivation by using visualization methods. Imagine attaining your objectives and experiencing the good sensations and results that come from making changes for the better.

It's crucial to keep in mind that changing your lifestyle takes time and that you will likely have setbacks along the way. As obstacles arise, it's critical to reassess objectives, look for assistance, and concentrate on implementing tiny, long-lasting adjustments. It is feasible to enhance heart health and general well-being by being motivated and dedicated to healthy adjustments.

Resources And Support Groups For Heart Disease In Males

For men with heart disease, support groups and services may be a great source of knowledge, emotional support, and useful guidance. People might feel less alone and better equipped to handle their illnesses by getting in touch with others who have gone through similar things.

The following organizations and resources might be beneficial for men with heart disease:

The American Heart Association (AHA) is a nonprofit group whose goal is to lower the incidence of heart disease and stroke. To promote heart health, they provide instructional materials, support networks, and advocacy initiatives.

A countrywide support system for people with heart disease and their families is called **Mended Hearts**. They provide support groups both offline and online, as well as instructional materials and advocacy initiatives.

WomenHeart: WomenHeart is a federal agency that focuses on female heart disease. Nonetheless, they provide tools and support groups that are also beneficial to males.

HeartSupport is an online community that offers information, support, and education to people with heart disease and their families.

Cardiac Rehabilitation Programs are systematic instruction and exercise plans that are often provided in hospitals and other healthcare facilities. These programs may provide guidance and instruction on managing medicine, stress, and lifestyle changes.

Resources For Mental Health: It's important to get assistance if necessary since mental health may play a significant role in the management of heart disease. The management of stress, anxiety, and depression may benefit from tools like therapy, counseling, and support groups.

Keep in mind that asking for help and resources is a show of strength, not weakness. Making connections with others who have gone through similar things may be a great source of knowledge, solace, and inspiration. Consider looking through these sites if you or a loved one is dealing with heart illness to get the help you need.

Techniques For Keeping An Optimistic Perspective

It may be difficult to have a good view of life, particularly while coping with health problems like heart disease. Yet it's crucial to have a positive outlook since it may enhance one's physical well-being and general quality of life. *These are some methods for keeping a cheerful view of life:*

One of the greatest strategies to maintain optimism is to **keep your attention on the present**. Concentrate on the now and what you can do to make your current position better rather than thinking about the past or the future.

Embrace thankfulness: It's possible to significantly enhance general well-being by practicing gratitude. Spend some time every day thinking about the blessings you have, such as excellent health, understanding friends and family, or a lovely day.

Discover your purpose and meaning in life: A feeling of satisfaction and a cheerful perspective may be attained by discovering your purpose and meaning in life. This may include participating in volunteer work, following a hobby or a passion, or making important objectives.

Be in touch with family and friends: Social support is crucial for sustaining a happy mindset. Try to keep in touch with your loved ones, whether it be by phone conversations, video chats, or in-person visits (when possible).

Take good care of your physical well-being since it's important for both. By maintaining a healthy lifestyle that includes a portion of nutritious food, enough rest, and frequent exercise, you may enhance your general well-being and keep a positive perspective.

Practice self-care: Making time for yourself and engaging in self-care activities will help you feel better overall and less stressed. This might be taking a soothing bath, reading a book, or engaging in yoga or meditation.

Get professional assistance: If you are having trouble keeping a positive mindset, it could be good to do so. A therapist, counselor, or another mental health specialist may be consulted in this regard.

It's crucial to keep in mind that keeping a good mindset does not entail rejecting or disregarding the difficulties that come with having heart disease. It's important to recognize and handle these difficulties while simultaneously emphasizing the good things in life. People with heart disease may retain a good perspective and enhance their general well-being by implementing these techniques into their everyday lives.

Conclusion

Millions of individuals throughout the globe suffer from heart disease, which is a significant and pervasive health problem. No of their age or origin, it is the biggest cause of mortality for males and may affect anybody. Yet, there is good news: early identification may save lives and heart disease is mostly avoidable. So, it is crucial to comprehend the causes, signs, and treatment options for heart disease.

We have looked at a variety of issues of male cardiac disease in this book. The risk factors for developing heart diseases, such as smoking, high blood pressure, high cholesterol, obesity, diabetes, and family history, have been covered in detail. Also, we have included advice on how to lower your chance of developing heart disease by making healthy lifestyle choices including quitting smoking, engaging in regular exercise, managing your stress, and eating a balanced diet.

The significance of understanding heart disease symptoms cannot be emphasized. Sadly, a lot of men put off going to the doctor until it is too late because they fail to notice the symptoms or are reluctant to confess to themselves or others that they may have a health problem. It is crucial to realize that treating heart disease effectively depends on early diagnosis. Men may dramatically increase their chances of survival and avoid long-term cardiac damage by detecting the signs and getting help right once.

Another crucial topic that we have covered in this book is heart disease prevention. Men may greatly lower their chance of developing heart disease by establishing good lifestyle practices. They include keeping a healthy weight, exercising often, eating a balanced diet, controlling existing medical disorders including high blood pressure, high cholesterol, and diabetes, and avoiding tobacco and excessive alcohol usage. While implementing these lifestyle adjustments might be difficult, doing so is essential for preserving excellent health and lowering the risk of heart disease.

Last but not least, it is critical to understand that heart disease is a complicated problem that requires a multifaceted strategy for prevention and treatment. To treat cardiac disease, medicine or surgery alone are insufficient. Instead, to properly treat and prevent heart disease, a comprehensive strategy that incorporates medication, medical procedures, and lifestyle changes is required.

Finally, the book Heart Disease in Men: Identifying the Signs and Lowering Your Risk offers crucial knowledge about the condition. To avoid heart disease, this book emphasizes the significance of identifying the warning symptoms, lowering risk factors, and establishing good lifestyle behaviors. Men may greatly increase their chances of enjoying a long and healthy life, free from the burden of heart disease, by following these guidelines. Never forget that it is never too late to begin caring for your heart health.